LIVING INSIDE THE
Health Matrix

Living Inside the Health Matrix

Why We Can't Stay Healthy Alone and What Truly Keeps Us Well

Tyler Yaqing Tang

TABLE OF CONTENTS

Introduction: Beyond Willpower—A New Framework for Health. 1

    Purpose and Vision 2

    What This Book Offers 4

Chapter 1: Seeing Our Health Through the Health Matrix 7

    The Three Dimensions of Health 8

    The Three Health Defenders 9

    The Health Matrix Framework 10

    Key Benefits of the Health Matrix 12

    Creating Health Equity and Innovation 14

    The Ultimate Vision 15

Chapter 2: The Three Dimensions of Health 17

    Understanding Each Health Dimension 18

    How the Three Dimensions Interact 24

    Achieving Health Balance 30

    Redefining Health for Modern Life 32

    Applying the Health Matrix to Your Life 33

    Moving Beyond Current Limitations 35

Chapter 3: The Three Health Defenders 39

    The Three Defenders of Our Health 40

    How the Three Defenders Work Together 46

    Principles of Effective Health Defense 47

    Practical Applications 50

    The Future of Health Defense 51

Chapter 4: Building a Healthier Life with the Health Matrix........ 55

    Life Transitions: Preparing for Change 56

    Detailed Case Study: Preventing Falls in Older Adults 58

    Adapting Health Priorities Across Life Stages 61

    Evaluating Activities Through the Health Matrix 63

    Practical Assessment Strategies 65

    Building Sustainable Health 66

Chapter 5: Toward More Equitable Health Access for All 69

    A Vision of True Health Equity 69

    Redefining Health Equity 70

    Health Rights for Vulnerable Populations 73

    Embracing Individual Differences 77

    Building Inclusive Systems 80

    Creating a Foundation for Human Flourishing 83

Conclusion... 87

Acknowledgements.. 91

About the Author... 93

INTRODUCTION

Beyond Willpower–A New Framework for Health

I F WE DON'T defend our health, we will ultimately lose it. We live in a world filled with health hazards that can compromise our well-being with or without our awareness: viruses and bacteria, natural disasters, accidents, long-term consumption of unhealthy substances, mental health challenges from prolonged screen time and social media, and the isolation that haunts so many of us. Sometimes we lose our health overnight from unexpected events; sometimes we lose it gradually.

To achieve optimal health, we must acquire knowledge, develop skills, and build habits to navigate various life circumstances. This means having the courage to say "no" to health hazards, foreseeing danger and taking precautions, becoming more disciplined, reaching out for help when needed, and sometimes facing our own fears and desires. In such a complex world, it's extremely difficult for anyone to consistently take the right steps and avoid harmful influences.

However, **relying on willpower alone to defend our health is unrealistic for most of us.** Willpower gets drained by demanding work, life burdens, and daily distractions. Many of us lack the mental energy to make rational health decisions consistently. The toxic environment we live in—expensive healthy groceries, easily accessible unhealthy food, addictive social media—makes staying healthy increasingly difficult. Even those who have strong willpower today shouldn't take it for granted. We were all once vulnerable children who didn't choose our circumstances, and we will all become vulnerable again before the end of our lives.

Health shouldn't be reserved only for those who are self-disciplined, have strong willpower, or have won the genetic lottery. All of us deserve a fair opportunity to improve our health with reasonable effort. As individuals, it's extremely difficult to navigate every aspect of our health throughout our dynamic life course. We need a comprehensive framework that factors in multiple dimensions of health and mobilizes both clinical and non-clinical people around us to help us stay healthy.

Purpose and Vision

This book introduces the **Health Matrix**—a framework that examines health through three key dimensions (physical, mental, and social) and identifies three types of health defenders who support us: doctors, interventionists, and health keepers. This matrix shifts healthcare from reactive problem-solving to proactive health-building, helping us identify root causes of preventable health issues and understand how our environment and relationships influence our well-being.

The Health Matrix empowers us to move beyond individual willpower by uniting multiple preventative care forces. Instead of doctors working alone, they collaborate with interventionists (who change our health trajectory through programs and environmental modifications) and health keepers (who help us maintain healthy habits and avoid hazards). When well-implemented, these three defenders work together to support long-term well-being without overwhelming reliance on personal discipline.

This book distinguishes itself through several key approaches:

Patient-Centered Focus: This framework is designed from the patient's perspective, and it thus prioritizes patient needs and desires as the catalyst for genuine health improvements. It's designed to benefit not only the educated and rational but also those in vulnerable positions—ensuring that next-generation preventative health leaves no one behind.

Framework Perspective: Rather than focusing on singular medical therapies or fitness programs, this book takes a broader view of preventative care, acknowledging that advancement requires attention to policies, incentive structures, delivery models, technologies, and cultural factors alongside medical services.

Innovation-Driven Future: This book is forward-looking, focused on immediate actions to shape better preventative health systems through collaboration among health professionals, scientists, technologists, policymakers, economists, and patients.

Equity and Inclusion: The framework addresses not only general population needs but also includes marginalized groups often overlooked by traditional healthcare—prisoners, refugees, homeless individuals, and others.

Enriched Medical Science: By incorporating data from daily activities and multiple perspectives, this framework will provide researchers with richer preventative health data, facilitating the generation of valuable medical knowledge.

What This Book Offers

The Health Matrix is for anyone interested in gaining a holistic understanding of health, including individuals, doctors, medical professionals, health innovators, technologists, economists, and regulators. Since health impacts everyone and we all have the potential to influence one another, I've minimized the use of jargon. While not everyone can become a doctor, everyone can play a role as an interventionist or health keeper for family, friends, and community members.

This framework advocates for integrating health considerations into every aspect of our lives and daily decisions while acknowledging the limitations of human nature. It redefines traditional roles: doctors become collaborative health steerers rather than isolated problem-solvers, fitness and wellness services are recognized for their medical value, and health keepers—those who maintain our daily well-being—receive the recognition and support they deserve.

The book envisions a future where preventative health is backed by scientific research that measures associations between specific services and health improvements, where innovation drives creative solutions, and where health equity ensures that everyone—regardless of demographics, career, or life experience—has access to comprehensive preventative care.

The Health Matrix does not attempt to negate or challenge the existing healthcare system. Instead, it focuses on how preventative healthcare can differentiate itself from and complement traditional medicine. It doesn't provide personal health advice or specific technological solutions—rather, it serves as a canvas for innovators to develop creative approaches that serve people worldwide.

The book begins with the Health Matrix framework, then explores the three health dimensions, three health defenders, and practical applications, concluding with how the Health Matrix ensures equitable access to health for everyone.

CHAPTER 1

Seeing Our Health Through the Health Matrix

T HE HEALTH MATRIX is a comprehensive framework that examines health through three key
dimensions—physical, mental, and social—and identifies
three types of health defenders who support us: doctors,
interventionists, and health keepers. This framework
shifts healthcare from reactive problem-solving to proactive health-building, empowering us to understand how
imbalances in one area can inhibit progress in another
and how targeted improvements can reinforce overall
wellness.

While many influential models have recognized the
interconnectedness of these health dimensions—from
the World Health Organization's definition of health as a
state of complete physical, mental, and social well-being
to George Engel's biopsychosocial model—the Health
Matrix offers a structured, dynamic approach that makes
these interactions both actionable and measurable. It's

designed not just for professionals but for anyone seeking integrated, practical ownership of their health.

The Three Dimensions of Health

To understand how the Health Matrix works, we must first examine the three fundamental dimensions that comprise human health. Each dimension represents a crucial aspect of our well-being, and optimal health requires attention to all three working in harmony.

Physical Health encompasses muscular strength, movement coordination, digestion, and sleep. A physically healthy person maintains a nutritious diet, exercises consistently, and carries out daily activities productively without developing preventable injuries or chronic conditions.

Mental Health relates to our cognitive abilities to recognize our capabilities, express emotions, and manage life stressors. A mentally healthy person uses their cognitive functions effectively without burning out their mental capacity.

Social Health refers to our ability to build healthy relationships with our environment and community. A socially healthy person builds rapport with others, addresses conflicts constructively, maintains balanced relationships, and can access social support when needed.

The Three Health Defenders

While understanding the three dimensions is important, achieving optimal health across all dimensions requires support from others. The Health Matrix identifies three types of people who serve as defenders of our health, each playing a distinct but complementary role in our wellness journey.

Doctors: The Health Steerers provide comprehensive medical knowledge and an objective view of our health needs. They engage in shared decision-making to establish short-term, mid-term, and long-term health goals. With access to our complete health picture—including medical records, activities, behaviors, living conditions, and relationships—they offer personalized preventative services and serve as our primary resource for health concerns, information, and recommendations.

Interventionists: The Change Leaders establish executable programs to actualize health goals identified by doctors. These programs range from nutrition management and exercise coaching to stress management and social engagement activities. They work in diverse settings—homes, gyms, parks, or virtual environments—delivering interventions that improve health across all three dimensions.

Health Keepers: The Health Maintainers ensure we

consistently engage in healthy behaviors and protect us from harmful actions. Their responsibilities range from preparing nutritious meals and serving as emergency contacts to accompanying us during health activities and helping us decline harmful choices. They make maintaining good health habits easier and more sustainable.

The Health Matrix Framework

Now that we understand the individual components, we can see how they work together in the complete Health Matrix system. This framework demonstrates the collaborative relationships between all three health defenders across all three health dimensions.

The Health Matrix shows how the three health defenders work collaboratively across the three health dimensions:

Health Defenders	Physical Health	Mental Health	Social Health
Doctors	• Assess nutrition, musculoskeletal health, living conditions • Recommend physical health intervention plans	• Evaluate cognitive habits, emotional patterns, and personality traits • Recommend stress management approaches	• Assess social relationships and networks • Recommend enhanced social engagement
Interventionists	• Provide nutrition plans and exercise coaching • Lead environmental changes • Implement health improvement programs	• Offer stress management programs • Provide mood regulation support	• Organize social engagement activities • Guide quality alone time
Health Keepers	• Ensure meal and exercise compliance • Prevent unhealthy patterns • Maintain hygiene and medication adherence	• Track stress levels • Provide protection from mental stressors	• Provide companionship and emotional support • Safeguard need for solitude

Figure 1: The Health Matrix

Key Benefits of the Health Matrix

Understanding how the Health Matrix works is just the beginning. The real value lies in the practical benefits this framework provides for individuals, healthcare providers, and society as a whole. These benefits demonstrate why this approach represents a significant advancement over traditional healthcare models.

From Reactive to Proactive Healthcare

Instead of viewing patients as collections of problems, the Health Matrix enables collaboration among all three defenders to identify opportunities for proactive health-building, even in the absence of illness. This approach breaks health improvements into actionable steps, allowing patients to make incremental changes that foster progress and achievement.

Multiple Access Points and Flexibility

Health journeys can begin anywhere within the nine boxes of the matrix, not just in doctors' offices. This flexibility makes it easier to identify improvements early while providing multiple types of support for implementation. Whether starting with an interventionist's program or a health keeper's daily support, all paths can lead to comprehensive wellness.

Comprehensive Problem-Solving and Gap Identification

The matrix reveals both existing health problems and gaps in support across all three dimensions. It identifies which defenders can address specific issues and helps doctors explore multiple factors contributing to health problems, particularly valuable for managing chronic illnesses and diseases with unknown causes.

Holistic Integration

By addressing physical, mental, and social well-being concurrently, the matrix ensures multiple factors are considered simultaneously. For example, when a patient experiences stressful life events, a doctor might initially recommend interventions targeting mental health (such as counseling) and social health (such as strengthening support networks), then evaluate progress over time.

Beyond Disease Prevention

The framework addresses not only clinical health issues but also quality-of-life questions: children's growth potential, hair loss concerns, the effects of high heels on posture, vision problems from screen time, and chronic stress management. When fully implemented, these issues could be addressed outside traditional clinical settings.

Clear Role Division and Continuous Improvement

The matrix clarifies each defender's responsibilities, making it easier to find the right support when changes are needed. It enables ongoing identification of improvement areas, allowing for consistent progress throughout one's lifetime and making health management a continuous process.

Creating Health Equity and Innovation

The Health Matrix encourages even distribution of medical resources across all three health dimensions and all three types of defenders, rather than concentrating primarily on doctors providing acute physical care. This includes supporting health keepers—often the most under-resourced defenders—who play crucial roles in maintaining wellness.

The framework aims to broaden health equity beyond universal coverage to include comprehensive preventative services for all population groups, especially those living on society's margins. By mobilizing traditionally non-medical professionals—nutritionists, fitness coaches, restaurants, gyms, and other businesses—into preventative health innovation networks, we can extend quality healthcare to every community.

Modern technology strengthens the Health Matrix by enabling more frequent health monitoring, expanding roles for all health defenders, fostering innovation in preventative health science, and creating new possibilities for population health improvement.

The Ultimate Vision

The Health Matrix enables people to achieve optimal health without needing to know everything about their health status. Through collaborative support from doctors, interventionists, and health keepers, even vulnerable individuals can become the healthiest versions of themselves.

For those living within this supportive framework, mental energy is freed for what matters most: enjoying life, pursuing happiness, achieving career success, and contributing meaningfully to the world. The matrix transforms health management from a burden into a foundation for human flourishing.

By shifting focus from "solving health problems" to "building health," the Health Matrix offers a roadmap for sustained wellness throughout life's transitions and challenges. When preventative and curative healthcare systems work seamlessly together, we can enter a new era of longer life expectancy, higher quality of life, and improved population health for all.

CHAPTER 2

The Three
Dimensions of Health

W E ACHIEVE OPTIMAL health when we reach a state of complete physical, mental, and social well-being. These three dimensions act like the legs of a tripod, collectively supporting our overall health. If one leg weakens or becomes disproportionately strong, the tripod cannot stand firmly, compromising our well-being. We can only achieve holistic health by viewing it through all three dimensions.

Understanding how physical, mental, and social health interact leads to greater overall well-being. When doctors grasp these interactions, they can identify root causes of many illnesses, treat patients more effectively, and prevent diseases before they manifest. Scientists can discover associations among these dimensions by studying them separately and together. Health policymakers who understand these interactions are more likely to enact legislation that promotes citizen health. This understanding empowers us to take better care of ourselves and our loved ones, make healthier choices in entertainment and travel, and navigate technological advances without compromising our well-being.

Understanding Each Health Dimension

To build a comprehensive understanding of the Health Matrix, we must first examine each dimension individually—exploring how they function, how they're currently addressed in healthcare, and why traditional approaches often fall short of optimal outcomes.

Physical Health: Beyond Absence of Disease

Physical health encompasses our body's strength, movement, energy, immune function, digestion, and overall ability to carry out daily activities without injury or disease. While modern medicine often focuses on treating physical symptoms—prescribing antibiotics for infections, chemotherapy for cancer, or medications for blood pressure—this approach works best when there's a single cause. However, many conditions result from multiple factors across all three health dimensions.

Consider high blood pressure, which can stem from physical factors (genetics, diet, lack of activity, alcohol consumption, and smoking), mental factors (chronic stress, anxiety, depression, and poor sleep quality), and social factors (work stress, social isolation, domestic violence, neighborhood safety, and cultural influences). When doctors only prescribe medication without addressing these underlying causes, patients often become dependent on drugs for life, missing opportunities to address manageable factors across all dimensions.

Relying solely on prescription drugs while ignoring other controllable physical, mental, and social aspects of illnesses results in many becoming dependent on medication, including those with initially mild conditions. This approach misses the opportunity to reverse manageable factors across the three health dimensions, leading to long-term medication dependence.

Unfortunately, most doctors do not address our physical, mental, and social well-being holistically in clinical settings. Their medical school training often doesn't cover conversations encompassing all three dimensions. Additionally, medical science doesn't always provide sufficient evidence to influence doctors' practices, and doctors aren't typically compensated for discussing all health factors affecting patients. Consequently, they often focus only on the most urgent manifested symptoms.

When doctors see us, they should look beyond just physical symptoms. The mere absence of physical symptoms is only a basic aspect of human health. Doctors should also pay attention to disease signs arising in patients' daily lives, assess manageable physical, mental, or social health factors contributing to issues, and consider our diet, exercise, work conditions, daily activities, emotional well-being, and relationships.

Mental Health: Moving Beyond Medication

Current medical practice often treats mental ailments like physical diseases, leading to overreliance on medication for mild issues. This reductionist approach fails to address the complex social and environmental factors that contribute to mental well-being.

When patients express mental health concerns, doctors frequently prescribe drugs to control symptoms, even when lifestyle changes—regular exercise, improved relationships, and reduced screen time—might resolve the underlying issues. For an adolescent experiencing school stress from excessive video game time, the first intervention should be working with parents to reduce screen time before prescribing drugs. Unfortunately, doctors rarely address underlying life circumstances causing mental distress.

The practice of labeling patients with mental disorders, even in mild cases, creates stigma that prevents people from seeking early help, allowing minor problems to develop into serious conditions. These days, guidelines doctors follow often involve labeling patients with various mental disorders. Even in mild and temporary cases, psychiatrists can find names to label patients. This labeling practice keeps many from seeking help at early stages. The stigma and knowledge that a mental disorder will be permanently recorded in medical records can scare patients away. As a result, they keep issues to themselves until minor problems grow into major health issues.

Many doctors are aware their practices need major changes, but they lack means to help patients beyond labeling them with mental diseases and treating them with prescription drugs. They often don't have resources to recommend exercise programs, social activities, or work with patients' families and friends to improve relationships. For doctors, prescribing drugs is the easiest way to help patients "feel better" immediately, but the side effects of mental health medications are apparent: patients become overly dependent on them.

The Health Matrix can serve as a roadmap to address this more effectively. When patients experience mild mental health issues, instead of prescribing drugs, doctors may assess the patient's physical, mental, and social health altogether, examining how they're doing with their interventionists and health keepers. Sometimes the root cause might derive from negligence by interventionists or health keepers—failure to engage patients in healthy social activities or overexposure to screen use. The root cause may also be stress from extensive mental activities like study and work without proper exercise and social activities.

Additionally, when patients are placed in the right environment or participate in suitable health intervention programs, their mental symptoms could resolve without psychiatric diagnosis. Doctors, interventionists, and health keepers could collectively provide a safe, private environment for patients with mild mental issues to heal through health intervention and health-keeping activities.

Social Health: The Overlooked Dimension

Social health—our ability to build healthy relationships and connect meaningfully with our environment—is often overlooked in clinical settings, yet many physical and mental health issues arise from social factors. The disconnection among physical, mental, and social health during clinical visits often leads doctors to overlook patients' social health factors, resulting in incomplete treatment approaches.

Consider athletes in competitive sports who endure chronic peer pressure and lack emotional support. To meet coaches' demanding requirements, athletes might overextend themselves in training, leading to depression from perfectionism and injuries from irrational risks. This issue is particularly prevalent in sports where athletes compete with high technical precision and lack collaborative peer relationships.

Even common social gatherings affect our health across dimensions. Family parties typically feature foods high in sugar, fat, and sodium, testing our willpower since most parties don't control portions. Consequently, physical health suffers. Many find social gatherings stressful due to comparisons based on appearance, wealth, and status. Consistently hearing ignorant comments from family and friends can accumulate into mental health issues. Not everyone feels connected at gatherings; some feel "left out" or "isolated" despite the seemingly fun environment.

We live in a society where the healthiest individuals are often the quietest. Those who go to bed early don't ask friends to sleep more when there's a spontaneous late-night food plan. The most disciplined aren't the most fun people in our social circles: when most party attendees are ready to get drunk, they leave quietly. When friends indulge in big barbecues, those cautious about their diet remain silent to avoid ruining the fun. Those who know how to protect themselves from bullying are reluctant to stand up for peers being bullied.

How the Three Dimensions Interact

Understanding the complex relationships among physical, mental, and social health is crucial for achieving optimal well-being. These interactions can be supportive, conflicting, or compensatory, and recognizing these patterns helps us develop more effective approaches to health maintenance and improvement.

Our physical, mental, and social well-being are intricately interconnected and influence one another in complex ways. Each dimension exists on its own spectrum—from low functioning (chronic illness, depression, and isolation) through middle ground (poor fitness, stress, and inconsistent connections) to high functioning (strength and vitality, emotional resilience, and meaningful relationships).

When Dimensions Support Each Other

Strong physical health brings energy that supports normal body and brain functioning, enabling us to carry out social activities, stay in good moods, perform well, boost confidence, and maintain close relationships. When our body is strong, we're more likely to carry out daily errands, strengthen our immune system, and reduce stress.

Good mental health helps us stay active, exercise regularly, improve sleep quality, and enhance communication skills to form stronger relationships. It promotes empathy and kindness, helping us build meaningful connections and stay optimistic about life's challenges.

Those with good social health receive high-quality health information that helps shape their lifestyle, engage in correct physical activities, and receive medical help when needed. Socially healthy people have trusted networks to reduce stress and anxiety, boost cognitive functions, and enjoy social bonds that encourage optimism and emotional resilience.

When Dimensions Conflict or Compensate

However, the relationship among the three dimensions isn't always harmonious. One dimension's strength can sometimes suppress others' development or mask underlying weaknesses in unexpected ways.

A person with strong social skills might consistently rely on others rather than developing physical or mental capabilities. This social reliance might be tolerated by those around them, but because of their strong ties, they miss opportunities to develop mental and physical health capabilities. If they suddenly lose social support, it becomes disastrous for their overall health.

Similarly, a technician may succeed at work through mental intelligence without tapping physical strengths or social skills. Such a work style could lead to chronic health issues if the technician doesn't exercise or improve their social life, ultimately representing a loss for them.

Sometimes strength in one dimension results from weakness in the other two, which can be counterintuitive. An antisocial person disconnected from social support might strive to work on physical and mental capabilities to build a "healthy image". While appearing healthy in both physical and mental dimensions, the disconnected social health may drive them to conduct antisocial activities destructive to others and themselves. Such weakness in one dimension is usually covered by dimensions that appear good.

Conversely, someone appearing physically weak might, thanks to mental clarity and social support, build an environment supporting their physical health and lead a life of longevity and health.

The "Second Gear" Problem: When Only Two Dimensions Function

Many of us live with two functioning health dimensions while lacking the third—a state that works temporarily but creates long-term vulnerabilities and anxiety. Our jobs, economics, and policies incentivize staying in this model without feeling setbacks. Many executives and leaders reach their positions by maintaining only two functional health dimensions.

Those lacking physical strength while being intelligent and kind constantly feel soft and vulnerable. After doing all the analysis and showing empathy, they cannot make things change for the better. Those with physical strength and mental sharpness likely lack empathy and social connectedness. As a result, their actions and speeches easily hurt others' feelings. Those with physical strength and social connectedness may lack intellectual capability to read scenarios and develop life solutions enhancing their well-being.

When two out of three health dimensions are thriving, we're likely to have achieved material needs, live well, have great careers, and play leadership roles in our communities. Incentives are low for achieving the third dimension we don't thrive in, especially since pursuing it could conflict with existing thriving dimensions.

For instance, a successful corporate leader with both physical strength and intelligence might find showing friendliness conflicts with his personal image. Efforts to show friendliness could make him and subordinates feel he's not genuine. Pursuing the third dimension could feel like self-betrayal, especially when he has already poured so much into building physical strength and intellectual mastery. Such feelings can stop him from achieving his better self.

The One-Dimension Trap

Making efforts on only one health dimension exposes us to serious long-term risks and issues. This narrow focus, while potentially creating short-term success, ultimately leaves us vulnerable to unexpected challenges and limits our overall potential for well-being.

Pursuing physical health extremely without tapping other dimensions may create a short-term healthy image. A person could lead a healthy physical life through nutritious food, physical activities, and good rest. However, lack of mental health pursuit prevents them from absorbing evolving health knowledge that could improve cognitive functions to combat uncertain health events. Meanwhile, lack of healthy social interactions makes it difficult to acquire latest health cautions from others and basic social support we all need. The only functioning dimension of physical strength could keep high-quality health information and helpful social networks at distance. Were any environmental changes or major life events to happen, physically healthy people could collapse from lack of social support and cognitive capabilities to cope with change.

Making efforts only on mental health may improve

cognitive functions, leading a person to understand health benefits and risks comprehensively. A mentally healthy person might be risk-averse and prevent many unnecessary known health risks like injuries, drowning, and accidents. However, due to lack of physical health pursuits, while acknowledging many health risks, they may lack strength to create change. Disconnection from healthy social networks makes acquiring high-quality health information time-consuming and tiring. The loneliness and anxiety from social disconnection could distort their ability to achieve well-being.

Those pursuing only social connectedness without improving physical strength and mental capabilities could become the "scapegoat" of their own life. Building relationships eagerly without strength leads to overcommitment and oversacrifice. There are always people who can "smell" our weakness and take advantage. Those overly committed in relationships without strength to say "no" or reject unreasonable requests could be victimized. Additionally, lack of cognitive capabilities to distinguish between genuine giving gestures and deceptive taking actions can easily "rip off" a person's energy from over-connectedness.

Achieving Health Balance

The pursuit of optimal health requires understanding both the tremendous challenges and profound rewards of integrating all three health dimensions. This integration represents perhaps the most difficult yet most rewarding path to lasting well-being.

The Difficulty and Reward of Integrating the Dimensions

Achieving all three health dimensions simultaneously is extremely difficult because it requires understanding their profound interactive effects, learning to balance competing forces, and adjusting to different life stages and scenarios. Physical efforts, thought processes, and social efforts must happen for us to understand ourselves. Obstacles exist everywhere in our living conditions, complex information sources, and emotions from people around us. These disturbing forces could cause us to lose balance among the three health dimensions at any point in our life course.

Yet achieving all three dimensions simultaneously is also the easiest way to live healthily. When we're ready to channel the three forces together to build healthy interactions with our surroundings, the world starts to reciprocate. When we present ourselves as living forms of strength, mental clarity, and kindness simultaneously, people can resonate with what a human being should be. Material resources, high-quality information, and social support start flowing to those capable of achieving this status. People can feel the difference we're making and the healthy influence we have on others. When we achieve all three health dimensions together, the wheel of our life starts turning for the better.

Building and Destroying Health

The asymmetry between building and destroying health reveals why sustained wellness requires such intentional effort and comprehensive approaches.

Destroying health is easy—harm any single dimension and overall well-being suffers. Even when only one health dimension is compromised and the other two remain functional, we cannot achieve complete well-being, and the compromised dimension will expose health issues over time.

But building health requires all three dimensions working concurrently and harmoniously over time. Building physical strength, improving mental sharpness, and enhancing social connectedness all require prolonged effort to see healthy results manifest. This is why sustained health is so challenging—the three dimensions must work together and need time to heal us and bring us to healthier lives.

Redefining Health for Modern Life

Our understanding of health must evolve to meet the demands of contemporary life, where traditional definitions of wellness prove insufficient for navigating complex, rapidly changing environments.

Understanding these interactive effects gives us a new definition of health: **our long-term optimal health can be achieved through our ability to adapt our physical, mental, and social health dimensions to the evolving environments we encounter throughout our life course.**

Different environments demand different emphases. In harsh conditions with scarce resources, physical capabilities may trump other dimensions for survival. In civilized worlds where foods are abundant and junk foods too accessible, our cognitive ability to be selective about food intake and make meaningful social connections with others becomes more important for thriving. In some tribal or sacred societies, residents' ability to build social bonds determines their access to food and supplies important for long-term health. In today's world, people immigrate more often than before, making our ability to adapt to new environments by applying all three health dimensions crucial for survival and prosperity.

When we're at the peak of physical, mental, and social well-being, we find it easy to exude strength, confidence, and attractiveness to others. At this stage, completing daily errands becomes easy; confronting work challenges becomes motivating; we speak with confidence and deliver messages precisely; exercise becomes enjoyment; making new friends and catching up with old ones becomes desirable; staying optimistic isn't difficult; and showing kindness and compassion becomes effortless. If we keep ourselves at this stage, we're likely to find our special meaning and purpose in life, become ready to help others with our unique capabilities, resist life distractions, and find our way back to the right track when things go wrong.

Applying the Health Matrix to Your Life

Understanding the three health dimensions theoretically is only the beginning; the real value lies in practical application. The following approaches can help individuals and healthcare providers implement this comprehensive framework effectively.

Visualization and Assessment

The first step in applying the Health Matrix involves creating a clear picture of current health status across all three dimensions. Doctors should visualize patients' current physical, mental, and social well-being to gain holistic understanding. This comprehensive evaluation helps identify potential improvements in each dimension and intertwined factors among them. For instance, a child with a single working parent may experience loneliness affecting social health, while the parent's busy schedule impacts the child's diet and physical health.

Since we became embryos, our parents have been planning our lives across all dimensions. They wish us to grow up healthy, intelligent, and have many good, supportive friends. This comprehensive approach should continue throughout our lives.

Developing Personalized Pathways

Once assessment is complete, the next step involves creating individualized approaches that respect each person's unique circumstances and capabilities. Every individual has unique combinations of health strengths and weaknesses. Doctors should co-develop personalized pathways to help people maximize all three dimensions. Some may need improvement in one or two areas, while others may need comprehensive enhancement. Some individuals in great shape simply need to maintain their health and continue thriving.

Tracking Progress Over Time

Sustainable health improvement requires consistent monitoring and adjustment of approaches based on observed outcomes. Health improvement takes days, weeks, months, and even years to show progress. After weeks of daily meditation programs, a patient may start enjoying occasional mental refreshment. After months of regular, structured exercise programs, stronger muscles become apparent. Sometimes recovery from traumatic brain events may take over a year.

Effective progress tracking helps both doctors and patients see the value of their efforts, make necessary adjustments, and stay motivated. Well-tracked progress also helps doctors and researchers understand benefits and effects of different preventative intervention programs on various patient groups, thereby continuously improving preventative care practice.

Moving Beyond Current Limitations

The current healthcare system, despite its many achievements, lacks the comprehensive approach necessary to address health through all three dimensions simultaneously. Recognizing these limitations is the first step toward developing more effective preventative care strategies.

The current healthcare system lacks means to help patients balance all three health dimensions effectively. The best mental therapy cannot fully aid a child constantly mistreated by parents. Enrolling a regularly mistreated girl in intervention programs believed to relieve stress but demanding hard work might only add pain to her life. She cannot simply meditate away social stress—her parents need help, not her.

To continuously improve preventative health services, doctors must gather high-quality data about how different health dimensions interact seamlessly, identify root causes before issues manifest, and collectively improve service quality to inspire a new generation of preventative health practice.

A doctor empowered to identify health risks across different dimensions early can provide long-term solutions to significantly minimize these risks for single parents and children. The doctor should "prescribe" combinations of programs and habit-change regimes helping parents and children improve all three well-being dimensions. These might include regular guided social events for children, low-cost meal plans with high nutritional value, and educational programs for both parents and children. This holistic approach helps them stay strong as families and mitigate risks associated with single-parent households.

This represents the future of preventative healthcare, where health is built proactively across all dimensions rather than reactively treating individual symptoms. When we understand and nurture all three health dimensions together, we create the foundation for lifelong wellness and the ability to adapt to whatever challenges life presents.

CHAPTER 3

The Three Health Defenders

MAINTAINING OPTIMAL WELL-BEING throughout our lifetime is both desirable and challenging. While we may achieve peak health during some prime years through individual effort, it's unrealistic to believe we can maintain this status independently across our entire life course. We all need help—sometimes continuous support. Even those who achieve optimal health during adulthood were once vulnerable children and will become vulnerable again as they age. We cannot escape our need for others to sustain our health.

Human beings' lack of willpower should not be the primary barrier to achieving optimal health. To thrive across all three health dimensions, we need collective efforts from three types of health defenders: doctors, interventionists, and health keepers. When these defenders collaborate seamlessly, our health thrives effortlessly. Without them, we rely solely on willpower to balance all dimensions—an approach that fails most of us.

The Three Defenders of Our Health

Doctors, interventionists, and health keepers act as three defenders of our health within the Health Matrix. Each plays a unique, irreplaceable role in helping us maintain wellness while collaborating to guard against preventable health issues. This framework provides an environment for them to cross-check each other's work, ensuring patients achieve optimal health without negligence or harm. Together, they deliver preventative care not only to those with strong wills but also to those who are vulnerable and need additional support.

Understanding these roles helps us clarify responsibilities; identify which defenders support us and which do not function effectively; pinpoint root causes of health issues; and find effective solutions. Importantly, collaboration among defenders is crucial—even if each performs optimally, isolation from one another can prevent us from achieving our best health outcomes.

Doctors: The Medical Stewards of Health

In an ideal preventative health practice, doctors provide regular medical support and knowledge beyond their traditional healthcare roles. They share responsibility for setting periodic health goals with us, using their comprehensive medical knowledge and independent stance to help us navigate health needs objectively and comprehensively.

Doctors serve as our primary resource whenever we have health concerns, seek information, or need assessments and recommendations. With access to our complete health picture—medical records, activities, behaviors, living conditions, and relationships—they offer preventative services tailored to our individual needs. They can treat us medically across all three health dimensions while also enhancing our overall health even when we are free from illness.

Holistic Health Guidance

Beyond medical treatment, doctors play a crucial role in optimizing our lives for maximum health benefits. With comprehensive knowledge of our health status, environment, lifestyle, and goals, they can predict our health trajectory and provide personalized recommendations. They should identify beneficial activities and encourage active engagement while helping us understand and avoid health risks.

Unlike traditional annual checkups, doctors in this framework see us more frequently to keep us on track, actively shaping our long-term health and well-being through guidance toward healthier trajectories, fostering better social connections, and recommending tailored activities.

Key Responsibilities

Doctors oversee our medical history and health status, making shared decisions about transitioning to healthier habits. This includes advising on what activities or behaviors to start or stop; providing resources to guide recommended changes; monitoring progress; and meeting regularly to reflect on improvements and adjust plans. Their medical expertise and comprehensive view are essential for effective health stewardship.

Interventionists: Masters of Health Change

Health interventionists excel at facilitating healthier transitions through structured programs that function like a doctor's toolbox. When doctors recommend behavioral changes, interventionists offer tailored programs to guide patients through these transitions. Their programs should be based on medical science with transparent designs, allowing doctors to understand operations and benefits confidently.

Interventionists develop and provide pre-approved health intervention programs; execute them in full compliance with doctors' requirements; and help patients thrive during the process. They track participation, commitment, and performance while completing the full program cycle from enrollment to feedback.

Evolution from Traditional Roles

Many traditional health professionals can evolve into interventionists:

Registered Dietitians and Nutritionists can establish engaging nutritional intervention programs, using their expertise to create effective diet change initiatives.

Occupational and Physical Therapists can adapt their skills to help patients develop healthy lifestyle skills and exercise programs for various patient groups.

Health and Exercise Coaches can enhance patients' holistic health through diet, addiction recovery, stress management, and fitness programs, providing ongoing support to achieve doctor-established goals.

Traditional Medicine Practitioners (Chinese medicine, Ayurveda, naturopathy, and homeopathy) can offer regimens that improve mood, sleep, pain relief, or boost resistance when integrated under the guidance of a doctor.

Collaborative Example

When a doctor determines an aging patient needs lower body muscle building to prevent falls, she refers the patient to an exercise coaching interventionist. The interventionist helps build muscles while tracking activities so the doctor knows exactly what the patient has undergone. This allows progress evaluation and further recommendations while keeping the doctor informed of potential issues and helping avoid risks.

Health Keepers: Guardians of Daily Wellness

While interventionists excel at motivating change, health keepers maintain the "status quo" of our well-being. They help us avoid cigarettes, alcohol, or drugs; monitor consumption of salt, sugar, or processed foods; ensure our living environment meets hygienic standards; and manage our social circles to prevent negative health influences.

Health keepers establish healthy living conditions and foster cultures that keep us away from health hazards. They know how to say "no" to us in loving, artful ways, making us feel cared for rather than offended. Even healthy adults need health keepers to maintain accountability and ensure compliance with doctors' and interventionists' guidance.

Examples of Health Keepers

Family members (parents, partners, and adult children) can be empowered with doctor and interventionist guidance to provide not just emotional support but tangible health improvements.

Close friends and relatives can serve as health keepers, especially for people living away from home; taking notes from doctors; ensuring medical guidance compliance; and participating in intervention programs.

Organizations and institutions can serve as health keepers:

- **Serviced apartments** offering healthy living conditions and exercise spaces
- **Schools** providing comprehensive health programs beyond basic education
- **Workplaces** ensuring safe, healthy environments with balanced job designs
- **Caregiving organizations** (orphanages and nursing homes) leveraging health resources for vulnerable populations

A Unique and Irreplaceable Role

Health keepers address questions seldom covered in doctors' offices. For young men worried about hair loss, health keepers can help build lifestyles that delay onset. For children with dust mite allergies, health keepers manage frequent bedding washing and house cleaning to improve living environments—tasks outside doctors' preventative care protocols.

Health keepers cannot be replaced by interventionists due to different timeframes and motivations. Interventionists work with patients for short periods, focusing on reaching specific milestones. Health keepers stay with patients for prolonged periods, maintaining stable states and "doing no harm." These different motivations require distinct skill sets: interventionists need motivational conversation skills, while health keepers need patience to avoid stimulating emotions.

How the Three Defenders Work Together

The interactive collaboration among defenders makes preventative health care more accessible and proactive with lower barriers. We can start our health journey with any defender—through health keepers who maintain our shape, interventionists like exercise coaches or nutritionists when we need help, or doctors for clinical visits. All paths can lead to comprehensive wellness.

This collaboration makes health improvement more proactive and effective, sometimes preventing health events before they occur. Health keepers who see us frequently can gather insights that help doctors identify improvement areas early, while interventionists can spot issues and share information with doctors during their work with us.

Patient-Centered Approach

The Health Matrix puts patients at the center of preventative care, with each defender providing one facet of service. Patients with the will to learn can acquire high-quality health knowledge from doctors, skills from interventionists,and hazard protection from health keepers. Together, the defenders help us see ourselves from 360 degrees, enabling us to stay healthy without unnecessary risks.

Each defender shows us different pieces of the health puzzle across the three dimensions. Doctors provide knowledge and fill gaps in our understanding; interventionists reveal what types of changes we handle well and which are difficult; health keepers expose our daily activities and patterns over time. This comprehensive view helps us learn what is best for ourselves while maintaining independence among defenders.

Principles of Effective Health Defense

Effective health defense rests on three principles: equal roles and collaboration among defenders, accountability and quality assurance mechanisms, and constructive conflict as a catalyst for growth.

Equal Roles and Collaboration

Doctors, interventionists, and health keepers share equivalent roles, departing from traditional healthcare where doctors dominate. This framework emphasizes equal participation, fostering intensive collaboration and communication. Empowering interventionists and health keepers enhances doctors' access to comprehensive patient information, enriching clinical decision-making capabilities.

The defenders ensure continuous health management, mitigating disruptions in preventative care. When one defender is unavailable, others can step in with established programs until replacement is found, ensuring seamless care transitions.

Accountability and Quality Assurance

The defenders assess each other's work and provide feedback to maintain superior care quality. If a patient with obesity resists a Mediterranean diet program, the health keeper can provide feedback to doctors, potentially leading to alternative programs that better accommodate patient preferences while maintaining health trajectories.

This inter-collaborative relationship allows continuous quality checks. Doctors receive feedback on how their decisions impact patient health over time; interventionists and doctors regularly check with health keepers to confirm correct protocol adherence; health keepers, who observe patients most closely, can identify issues in doctors' decision-making or interventionists' activities.

Constructive Conflict and Growth

The defenders are not expected to function in harmony at all times. Driven by different values, incentives, and skill sets, conflicts may arise—and these can be healthy when all prioritize patient health. Creative resolutions from conflicts help defenders grow perspectives, sharpen skills, and enrich experience, often improving patient health outcomes.

Doctors, interventionists, and health keepers should be able to criticize each other's decisions constructively. Doctors develop comprehensive medical understanding; interventionists know how patients perform in practice and may identify blind spots; health keepers spend the most time with patients and may spot irrationalities in decisions or activities.

Practical Applications

The Health Matrix has three main areas of practical application: preventing medication errors through collaborative oversight, moving patients beyond binary thinking about health choices, and creating supportive environments that reduce reliance on willpower alone.

Preventing Medication Errors

The collaborative efforts among defenders create a safety net preventing medication errors throughout prescribing, dispensing, and administering processes. Pharmacists (as interventionists) and health keepers can review prescriptions and raise questions about suspicious orders. Health keepers ensure correct drug dispensing when picking up medications and proper administration while monitoring patient reactions and adherence.

This collaboration reduces reliance on patient willpower alone to comply with prescriptions correctly. The delivery model mobilizing all three defenders potentially outperforms traditional approaches where patients rely solely on self-discipline and attention to detail.

Moving Beyond Binary Thinking

Many health challenges stem from binary thinking—smokers debating whether to have the next cigarette; drinkers questioning whether to drink; people struggling with whether to eat unhealthy foods. This binary thinking strains willpower and often leads to giving in to unhealthy behaviors.

The three health defenders can help patients reach a third mental state: "it didn't occur to me at all." When patients stop thinking about whether they should engage in harmful behaviors, they're more likely to abstain because their focus shifts elsewhere.

Example: Reducing Sugar Consumption

For a patient who consumes too much sugar daily, doctors set goals to cut sugary food intake; interventionists develop appealing yet healthy meal plans and engaging weight management programs; while health keepers remove sweet foods from work and home environments and engage patients in enjoyable activities. This collective effort builds a microenvironment where patients do not face constant binary decisions about consuming sweets, freeing them from the dilemma over time.

The Future of Health Defense

Two key considerations will shape the implementation of health defense: ensuring fair recognition and rewards for all defenders, and understanding the limitations of having one person or organization serve all three defender roles.

Fair Recognition and Rewards

All three defenders should receive fair recognition for their health enhancement efforts. Doctors contribute expertise for high-quality shared decisions; intervention-ists bring specific skill sets; health keepers offer time, attention, and intensive labor. The proportion of recogni-tion may vary based on circumstances—minimal health keeper roles for healthy adults versus intensive commit-ment for disabled patients requiring daycare.

Limitations of Single-Entity Defense

While theoretically possible for one entity to serve all three defender roles, this approach has significant limi-tations. A parent serving as doctor, interventionist, and health keeper for their children raises questions about time availability, objectivity, and potential stress creation. Similarly, nursing homes acting as all three defenders for elderly residents face conflicts of interest that could harm patients. Therefore, maintaining separate entities for each defender role provides necessary checks and balances for optimal patient care.

The Health Matrix framework recognizes that optimal health requires collaborative support beyond individual willpower. By clearly defining roles, fostering collaboration, and maintaining accountability among doctors, interventionists, and health keepers, we create a comprehensive system that makes sustained wellness achievable for everyone, regardless of their personal discipline or circumstances.

CHAPTER 4

Building a Healthier Life with the Health Matrix

T HE HEALTH MATRIX serves as both a diagnostic tool and a roadmap for building healthier lives across different circumstances and life stages. By examining our health through the lens of three dimensions and three defenders, we can identify missing pieces, prioritize our efforts, and adapt to changing needs over time. This chapter explores how to apply the Health Matrix practically through key life scenarios, demonstrating how the framework guides us toward optimal health with minimum effort.

Rather than relying solely on willpower or accepting health as predetermined, the Health Matrix helps us systematically address health challenges by breaking them into manageable components and mobilizing appropriate support systems.

Life Transitions: Preparing for Change

One of the most challenging aspects of maintaining health occurs during major life transitions. The Health Matrix provides a valuable framework for navigating these changes by helping us prepare systematically rather than relying on chance or individual resilience alone.

The Fish Tank Principle

Experienced fish owners know that when changing water for their fish, they should keep some original water in the tank before adding new water. This prevents abrupt environmental changes and helps fish adapt more easily, diluting potential harm from water that might be too hot or cold.

Human beings face similar challenges during major life transitions—going to college, getting married, starting new jobs, or moving to new homes. While these changes are generally positive, many people ignore the sudden environmental shifts they create. Mental health issues are prevalent in universities; divorce rates remain high; people complain about negative health impacts from sedentary jobs, workplace pressure, and office politics. These life events, while appearing beneficial from the outside, often come with hidden costs because people enter new situations without adequate preparation or experience.

Applying the Health Matrix to Transitions

The Health Matrix transforms how we approach major life changes by enabling systematic preparation across all three health dimensions before transitions occur.

Consider an eighteen-year-old student finishing high school and moving to college. They must adjust to a new city, lose access to familiar support systems, disconnect from family and friends, and adapt their diet, sleep patterns, exercise routines, and social connections while managing academic demands. This complete lifestyle turnover creates tremendous pressure, with physical, mental, and social health foundations suddenly disrupted.

Using the Health Matrix perspective, students can better prepare for college during high school when families can work on developing adaptive capabilities across all three dimensions. Parents can prepare children for social independence by involving them in intervention programs that expose them to new friends and environments. They can develop meal preparation skills for independent living and gradually increase autonomy in decision-making. These interventions across physical and social health dimensions can happen well before college begins, so students arrive better equipped to handle environmental changes while focusing on intellectual growth.

This approach transforms students from fish suddenly thrown into a new tank to individuals chronically exposed and adapted to new environments, reducing health risks and increasing chances of thriving in their chosen paths.

Detailed Case Study: Preventing Falls in Older Adults

To illustrate how the Health Matrix functions in practice, the following case study demonstrates comprehensive preventative care coordination among all three health defenders across multiple health dimensions.

Nancy's Comprehensive Care

A geriatrician determines that fifty-five-year-old Nancy faces increasing fall risk after diagnosing early-stage osteoporosis through a dual X-ray absorptiometry (DEXA) scan. Gait, balance, and functional tests confirm moderate fall risk despite early-stage osteoporosis diagnosed through DEXA. Rather than immediately prescribing denosumab (an injectable medication that is hard to stop due to rapid bone loss after discontinuation, hence not ideal early on), the doctor recommends alendronate (a weekly oral tablet that can be discontinued if bone health stabilizes) plus vitamin D3 supplements. The doctor then refers Nancy to various interventionists who meet regulatory standards for fall prevention through education, nutrition, exercise, and environmental modifications.

Educational Intervention: Nancy joins an online in-network educator for fall prevention classes. She learns about multiple contributing factors to falls at her age and the importance of leg strengthening to prevent muscle loss. The educator teaches that most elder falls occur in bathrooms, making environmental improvements crucial. Nancy replaces old slippers with non-slip versions and receives certification of completion in her health records.

Nutritional Intervention: Nancy increases calcium-rich foods in her diet. Her local supermarket, part of the healthcare network, provides an on-site registered dietitian who helps Nancy shop for appropriate food combinations. She incorporates more dairy products, leafy greens like kale and turnip greens, and protein sources including lean meats, legumes, and eggs. With Nancy's consent, her shopping records connect to her electronic health records.

Exercise Intervention: Nancy joins exercise intervention classes at a local gym certified to provide fall prevention programs. The coach teaches her gait, balance, and functional training through muscle strengthening exercises such as chair-assisted movements, squats, and stability exercises. Each session is recorded in Nancy's health records with performance evaluations.

Environmental Intervention: Nancy works with a company specializing in home environment evaluation and fall-prevention equipment installation. They identify missing bathroom safety equipment—grab bars around the shower, shower chairs, and non-slip mats—and install them properly, reporting modifications to Nancy's doctor through her health record system.

Health Keeper Role: Nancy's son who lives with her serves as her health keeper. After several weeks of gym training, both Nancy and her coach believe she can confidently perform exercises at home. The coach authorizes Nancy's son to monitor her home exercise activities, following specific instructions for performance evaluation and ensuring daily adherence. The son and coach maintain periodic contact to ensure proper completion of recommended tasks, even during travel.

Integrated Results: With Nancy's consent, her doctor accesses records of class attendance, exercise participation, and environmental modifications. Any adherence issues prompt alternative recommendations. During quarterly visits, the doctor conducts follow-up tests showing improvements in gait, balance, and function. After three years of follow-up, Nancy's periodic DEXA scans show that her fall risk has settled at a low level, and the doctor discontinues medication, providing a "medication vacation" due to her stabilized medical status.

Adapting Health Priorities Across Life Stages

Our health needs evolve continuously throughout our lives, requiring different emphases and approaches at various developmental stages. The Health Matrix supports these natural transitions by providing a flexible framework that can be adapted to focus on the most critical areas while maintaining comprehensive support.

The Dynamic Health Matrix

Throughout our lifetime, we must shift focus among health priorities based on developmental needs and circumstances. The Health Matrix supports these transitions by allowing us to emphasize different combinations of dimensions and defenders while maintaining overall balance.

Infancy and Early Childhood: Newborn infants primarily need physical health attention for safety and healthy development. The health keeper-physical health combination takes center stage, with doctors and interventionists playing supporting roles through counseling parents and providing necessary interventions. Mental and social health development becomes more prominent as children grow into toddlers and adolescents.

Adolescence: A teenage boy entering adolescence may need primary focus on healthy mental development, with intensive interventions through exercise and social activities. The interventionist-mental health combination moves to the center, while parents (health keepers) play supportive roles by facilitating program participation and learning when to step back during emotional disturbances. Professional interventionists handle sensitive developmental challenges while parents maintain positive relationships by avoiding untrained intervention during conflicts.

Adulthood: Healthy adults may need balanced attention across all dimensions, with emphasis shifting based on life circumstances—career demands, family responsibilities, or health challenges that emerge over time.

This dynamic approach allows patients and health defenders to allocate resources wisely, focusing on the most critical areas while maintaining support across all dimensions.

Evaluating Activities Through the Health Matrix

Beyond managing transitions and life stages, the Health Matrix serves as a powerful tool for evaluating the health benefits of various activities and relationships. This systematic approach helps us make informed decisions about how we spend our time and energy.

Sports and Recreation Assessment

The Health Matrix provides an excellent framework for evaluating the health benefits of various activities. Breaking down benefits into physical, mental, and social dimensions helps us understand whether activities serve our comprehensive health needs.

Example: Sailing provides physical benefits through rigging, de-rigging, and crew movements required for boat balance and rope handling. Mental benefits include reading wind direction, coordinating multiple variables for navigation, and strategic planning to maximize wind power. Social benefits emerge through crew coordination and weekend activities with friends. This analysis reveals sailing as a sport that effectively addresses all three health dimensions.

Example: Swimming offers excellent physical strength building but limited social interaction due to its individual nature. Swimmers might need to seek social health development outside the pool through other activities or group swimming programs.

This systematic evaluation helps us make informed choices about recreational activities, avoid poorly designed sports that create injury risks, and potentially inspire new activities that address multiple health dimensions simultaneously.

Relationship Dynamics

The Health Matrix framework extends beyond individual health to guide the development and maintenance of healthy relationships throughout various life circumstances.

The Health Matrix also guides healthy relationship development. When couples marry, they can identify each other's roles in their partner's health: one partner skilled in sports might serve as a physical health keeper for the other; one with strong social skills might be a social health keeper for a more introverted partner. Clear identification of characteristics using the Health Matrix can improve post-marriage quality of life and guide creation of nurturing environments for children.

Even during divorce, the Health Matrix can minimize damage to all parties. A mother who has served as the children's physical health keeper through sports activities might continue in that role; a father gaining custody might develop health keeper skills across all dimensions while still coordinating with the mother for sports and social activities. This approach maintains children's health matrix integrity while minimizing health impacts during family transitions.

Practical Assessment Strategies

Moving from theoretical understanding to practical implementation requires concrete strategies for evaluating our current health status and identifying areas for improvement. The following approaches provide systematic methods for applying the Health Matrix to personal health assessment.

Four Key Evaluation Areas

1. **Identifying Neglected Health Dimensions:** Determine if any of the three health dimensions are being ignored in daily life. Short-term neglect may not show immediate effects, but long-term ignorance of one dimension creates accumulating health risks. An office worker sitting for extended periods may maintain mental acuity and workplace relationships but face predictable spinal issues without physical exercise intervention.

2. **Determining Needed Defenders:** Identify which defenders are most needed for specific health

improvements. Sometimes we need doctors for thorough health evaluation and feedback; sometimes interventionists can address poor diet, exercise routines, or stress management; sometimes health keepers can guard against health hazards. The Health Matrix helps identify whose help should be central for particular preventative needs.

3. **Assessing Resource Allocation:** Evaluate whether time and effort are proportionally distributed among dimensions and defenders. Overreliance on one dimension or defender can create long-term health issues. For instance, relying solely on doctors without interventionist and health keeper support often leads to poor adherence and suboptimal outcomes.

4. **Evaluating Coordination:** Assess how well the three defenders coordinate to deliver health across all dimensions. This comprehensive view identifies weak links in collaboration and potential synergies that achieve optimal health outcomes with minimum effort.

Building Sustainable Health

The Health Matrix provides a framework for exploring life opportunities without sacrificing health. Many people achieve success without compromising ethical values, live happily without harming others, and gain freedom without unnecessary sacrifices. By maintaining health as a consistent factor in life decisions, supported by coordinated efforts among doctors, interventionists, and health keepers, individuals can live life to the maximum while achieving longevity with high quality of life.

This systematic approach transforms health from a constraint on life choices into an enabling framework that supports whatever paths we choose to pursue. Whether navigating major transitions, managing ongoing health needs, or optimizing daily activities, the Health Matrix provides the structure and support necessary for sustained wellness across all dimensions of human health.

CHAPTER 5

Toward More Equitable Health Access for All

T RUE HEALTH EQUITY requires more than equal access to healthcare; it demands systems that embrace human diversity while ensuring everyone can achieve their optimal health potential across all three dimensions.

A Vision of True Health Equity

In a healthier world built on true equity and embracing of human diversity, health outcomes would not be predetermined by circumstances of birth, geography, or social position. This vision extends far beyond traditional healthcare access to encompass comprehensive preventative health opportunities for all people, regardless of their background, circumstances, or life choices.

Infants born in the most rural areas would have comparable life expectancy with those born in the most prosperous cities. Children growing up in orphanages would expect to live healthy lives just like those brought up by both parents. Manual workers could carry out their work with minimum health risks, similar to nonmanual laborers. The uneducated population would have access to support systems guiding them to make informed health decisions just like the well-educated. Refugees would have equal access to living conditions that promote safety and health, similar to lawful citizens. Individuals of different sexual orientations could reach similar life expectancies while leading diverse lifestyles. One's level of wealth would not necessarily predict their maximum potential age, and differences in skin color would not indicate differences in life span.

This chapter explores how the Health Matrix framework can help us achieve this vision by redefining health equity, addressing the needs of vulnerable populations, embracing individual differences, and building truly inclusive preventative health systems.

Redefining Health Equity

Traditional approaches to health equity have focused primarily on equal access to healthcare services when people become sick. While important, this reactive approach fails to address the fundamental inequities that determine whether people stay healthy in the first place. True health equity requires a fundamental shift toward preventative health systems that recognize and address the full spectrum of factors affecting human wellness.

Beyond the "Winner Takes All" Culture

In politics, business, entertainment, sports, education, and other contemporary industries, the culture of "winner takes all" prevails. This system maximizes individual potential and rewards top performers but often wastes talent and overlooks those with minor "flaws." While this approach may work in competitive industries, it fundamentally conflicts with the nature of health and wellness.

The future preventative health system must defy this "winner takes all" culture for several crucial reasons. Every individual's health status is unique—our genetic composition, upbringing, meals, sleep patterns, education, work style, and lifestyles are all distinct. We follow our own paths of growth, maturity, and aging while battling different environments and personal challenges. No one should be rewarded simply for being healthier than others; we are our own allies and enemies in the health journey.

All efforts to enhance one's health should count and be recognized. Unlike other industries where people are not rewarded during training periods, the preventative health system must provide recognition and support for every step toward better health. Regardless of age, gender, job nature, geographic location, ethnic background, country of residence, immigration status, sexual orientation, or even imprisonment status, people should be able to connect and participate in the health system. When patients feel the need to connect or reconnect with preventative health support, they should always find the platform accessible and earn recognition for their efforts.

Expanding the Definition of Health Rights

Current definitions of health equity such as "equal access to health care services" and "equal opportunities for achieving full potential for health and well-being", while valuable, remain insufficient for true transformation. These definitions focus primarily on access to treatment rather than comprehensive support for achieving optimal health. True health equity must encompass equal access to preventative health programs that help people achieve and maintain optimal health, equal potential for earning "health wealth" through participation in wellness activities, equal opportunities to address intrinsic health risks, and equal rights to policy considerations based on scientific evidence from preventative health systems.

When we view health through the three dimensions—physical, mental, and social—the definition of health equity naturally evolves. Everyone should be entitled to access health services that optimize their potential across all three dimensions. Throughout our lifetimes, everyone should feel entitled to reach the optimum status of their physical strength, mental clarity, and social connection. Only when we reach our optimal status can we discover who we are, what our life mission is, what we care about, and how to love those around us.

Health Rights for Vulnerable Populations

Vulnerable populations face unique challenges that require specialized approaches within the Health Matrix framework. Rather than viewing these groups as problems to be solved, we must recognize them as individuals deserving equal access to health optimization, regardless of their circumstances or choices.

Advancing Rights for Incarcerated Individuals

In the United States, prisoners sentenced to life in prison are estimated to have an average life expectancy that is ten years shorter than that of civilians. This reduced lifespan results not only from mental status and physical conditions but also from poor living conditions in most penitentiary systems. As Alexander Paterson, a prison commissioner in the 1920s stated, people "come to prison as punishment, not for punishment." Yet current statistics do not reflect this principle.

The future preventative health system must support

prisoners' health needs proactively. When preventative health researchers identify benefits of specific intervention programs for inmates, the system should grant access to legitimate programs. For example, if daily thirty-minute guided meditation programs prove to reduce mental health issues for inmates, all prisons should make such programs accessible. Inmates should have freedom to participate in evidence-based health programs while serving their sentences.

When it comes to the three health defender roles, correctional facilities should act as health keepers, ensuring that inmates' physical, mental, and social health do not deteriorate during detention. This includes access to nutrition management programs, exercise training, mental health maintenance, and social programs. Since jails and prisons limit access to outside information and social connections, they bear responsibility for maintaining healthy environments and preventing isolation-related mental health problems.

Supporting Sex Workers' Health and Safety

Internationally, almost no countries have successfully eradicated prostitution. Some countries have legalized or decriminalized sex work, yet sex workers continue to suffer from discrimination, violence, and legal consequences that deteriorate their health. Their health rights cannot be effectively protected under most legal frameworks worldwide.

The preventative health system can support this population in multiple ways. Sex workers should learn how to carry out their work with minimum health risks, practice saying "no" to dangerous requests, and receive regular health screenings. Different from traditional screening approaches, sex workers could be rewarded for maintaining clean health records, with each effort to minimize risks counted through incentive mechanisms.

For those who not only minimize their own health risks but also help educate peers about health management, the preventative health system could create career pathways allowing transition to sexual health intervention program providers or caregivers. Their experience could help vulnerable individuals in the industry stay healthy and minimize risks to the greatest extent possible.

The system should also help sex workers maintain connections with society through social groups or online communities that protect their identity and privacy. Mental health support should help them develop clear divisions between "work" and personal life, minimizing job-related health impacts.

Protecting Refugee Health During Transitions

Refugees face unique preventative health challenges. Many flee their countries in relatively good health but encounter tremendous stress on their physical, mental, and social well-being during transitions. These health needs cannot be addressed solely through insurance coverage or basic humanitarian aid.

The uncertainty refugees face can bring mental health issues such as stress and insomnia. Without intervention, these problems can develop into advanced conditions over time. Refugees may also face shortages of high-quality food, depriving them of necessary nutrition long-term. Socially, many have lost close family and friends, making it difficult to form new relationships and participate in healthy social activities.

An established preventative care system should support refugees through transition periods with language classes, social activities, stress management courses, nutritional support, and exercise programs. These interventions can prevent health disadvantages while helping refugees become productive members of their new communities and reducing burden on hosting countries' healthcare systems. The goal is helping refugees become increasingly independent from a health perspective while maintaining their dignity and cultural identity.

Embracing Individual Differences

No two individuals are alike in their health needs, circumstances, or optimal pathways to wellness. A truly effective preventative health system must recognize and celebrate this diversity while ensuring equitable access to appropriate support for all people.

Developing Personalized Pathways

Every individual possesses a unique combination of health strengths and weaknesses shaped by genetics, environment, experiences, and personal preferences. The personalized preventative health system must empower health professionals to co-develop individualized pathways that help each person maximize their physical, mental, and social health potential.

Some patients may face acute needs in specific health dimensions, while others require chronic improvements across all three areas. Still others may already maintain good health across all dimensions and simply need programs to maintain and enhance their well-being. The system must be flexible enough to meet people wherever they are in their health journey and provide appropriate support for their next steps.

This personalization extends beyond medical interventions to encompass cultural preferences, lifestyle constraints, economic circumstances, and personal values. A preventative health approach for a rural farmer will necessarily differ from one designed for an urban professional, just as approaches for recent immigrants will differ from those for established community members.

Tracking Progress Across Diverse Populations

"Rome wasn't built in a day"—and neither is optimal health. It takes weeks, months, and even years for patients to see progress in their health improvements. After weeks of participating in daily meditation programs, a patient may start to enjoy occasional mental refreshment. After months of regular, structured exercise programs, they may feel stronger muscles. Recovery from traumatic events may take over a year to manifest meaningful progress.

Effective progress tracking must account for these varied timelines while helping both health defenders and patients recognize the value of their efforts, make necessary adjustments, and maintain motivation throughout the process. Well-tracked progress also helps doctors and researchers learn about the benefits and effects of different preventative intervention programs on various patient groups, enabling continuous improvement in preventative care practices.

The tracking system must be sensitive to cultural differences in how progress is measured and valued. Some cultures emphasize individual achievement, while others prioritize community well-being. Some focus on physical metrics, while others value spiritual or emotional growth. The system must accommodate these differences while maintaining scientific rigor and evidence-based approaches.

Recognizing Diverse Approaches to Health

People naturally gravitate toward different approaches to health and wellness based on their personalities, experiences, and circumstances. Some individuals thrive with structured, goal-oriented programs, while others prefer flexible, intuitive approaches. Some respond well to group activities and social support, while others prefer private, individual interventions.

The Health Matrix framework accommodates this diversity by recognizing that there are multiple valid pathways to optimal health across the three dimensions. Whether someone achieves physical fitness through traditional exercise, dance, martial arts, or manual labor matters less than their overall physical well-being. Similarly, mental health can be supported through therapy, meditation, creative expression, intellectual pursuits, or spiritual practices.

This recognition of diverse approaches extends to cultural and traditional healing practices. While maintaining scientific standards for safety and efficacy, the system should remain open to incorporating valuable insights from various healing traditions, recognizing that different approaches may work better for different populations.

Building Inclusive Systems

Creating truly equitable preventative health systems requires intentional design that considers the full spectrum of human diversity and circumstances. This involves not only removing barriers to access but actively creating pathways that work for all people, regardless of their starting point or life situation.

Considerations for System Design

When building preventative health delivery systems, we must ensure that patients from diverse population groups can benefit equally from available services. A patient shopping in high-end supermarkets and one shopping at farmer's markets should both access foods that provide necessary nutrition. Those who exercise at luxury gyms and those who exercise at home with simple equipment should achieve similar musculoskeletal health benefits. Those embracing technology in daily life should enjoy similar life expectancy with those who prefer life closer to nature.

The Health Matrix framework makes this equality possible while embracing diversity. The three health defenders—doctors, interventionists, and health keepers—can be individuals, non-profit organizations, or for-profit companies. Patients should be able to thrive regardless of the delivery model of their health support system, whether through high-tech solutions or community-based approaches.

A functioning preventative health system must provide infrastructure that assists policymakers with evidence while guaranteeing that different population groups are legally protected in accessing preventative health services tailored to their individual needs. These groups should be legally entitled to extensive preventative care interventions ensuring they can achieve optimal health status equivalent to any other population.

Adapting to Different Cultural Contexts

The implementation of preventative health systems must be sensitive to cultural, geographic, and economic contexts while maintaining core principles of equity and effectiveness. In the United States, the system should balance freedom, happiness, and health by providing services that enable patients to visualize their health and see benefits or risks of lifestyle choices without intruding on personal freedom.

In countries with universal healthcare like the United Kingdom and Germany, the challenge lies in extending comprehensive preventative services beyond current treatment-focused models while addressing resource constraints and ensuring equitable access across urban and rural populations.

In countries like China, where traditional medicine is integrated with Western medicine approaches, the system must respectfully incorporate valuable traditional practices while maintaining scientific standards for safety and efficacy. This requires ongoing research and dialogue between traditional practitioners and modern health professionals.

Addressing Global Health Challenges

Even in extreme circumstances such as war zones, the preventative health system must strive to maintain human dignity and health rights. While basic needs like food, water, and shelter are essential, people in affected areas also need access to mental health support and social connection services to help them rebuild their lives.

The preventative health framework can guide the management of refugee camps, detention centers, and other institutional settings where people's freedom is restricted. In these situations, the institutions act as health keepers with responsibility for maintaining residents' physical, mental, and social well-being. Independent doctors and interventionists should provide services to ensure accountability and prevent neglect or abuse.

Creating a Foundation for Human Flourishing

The ultimate goal of equitable, diverse preventative health systems extends beyond individual wellness to create conditions for human flourishing at all levels of society. When we achieve our optimal health status across all three dimensions, we become more likely to appreciate our genetic differences, accept diversity among people, and show empathy for others' unique strengths and limitations.

The Interconnection of Health and Social Progress

Only when we achieve balance across the three health dimensions with support from all health defenders can we learn about ourselves and our lives thoroughly. We can live in different lifestyles and exist in different forms while knowing we share the same platform when it comes to health. This shared foundation enables us to understand each other more clearly, show genuine empathy, and work together on shared human missions.

True health equity creates a foundation for addressing

other social challenges. When people's basic health needs are met and they have pathways to optimize their well-being, they are better equipped to contribute to their communities, pursue education and meaningful work, build healthy relationships, and engage in civic life.

Moving Forward Together

The vision of health equity and embracing diversity outlined in this chapter requires sustained commitment from individuals, communities, organizations, and governments. It demands that we move beyond traditional approaches that treat symptoms to comprehensive systems that address root causes and support human potential.

This transformation will not happen overnight, but each step toward more equitable, inclusive preventative health systems brings us closer to a world where everyone can achieve their optimal health potential. By embracing both our shared humanity and our individual differences, we create conditions for a healthier, more just world for all people.

The Health Matrix framework provides a roadmap for this transformation, offering practical tools for understanding health holistically while ensuring that no one is left behind. As we move forward, we must remain committed to the principle that health is a fundamental right that belongs to all people, regardless of their circumstances, choices, or starting point in life.

CONCLUSION

WE ARE ALL entitled to maximize the power of our physical, mental, and social health dimensions throughout our lives. We are all entitled to find the balance of our three health dimensions on our own terms. And we are all entitled to access the support we need to optimize those three health dimensions.

Health, just like freedom and happiness, is so crucial yet so different for all of us. We all have the equal right to achieve optimal health through the lens of the three health dimensions. We all share the same pursuit of health, yet as individuals, we might define our health differently. When we're able to achieve our own version of optimal health, we can live a life that is uniquely satisfying to us.

Understanding the interactive effects of the three health dimensions will help us identify potential health risks and issues early on, address them before they escalate, and work to continuously balance our physical, mental, and social health needs. We should not see the three health dimensions as independent influences on our health. Learning how they support and inhibit each other can help us identify the root causes of many health issues that often go unnoticed. This multidimensional view allows us to see ourselves as individuals with unique health needs—and to achieve wellbeing in our own way.

In our pursuit of health, we will make many mistakes—derail from healthy diets, skip important exercise, expose ourselves to distractions, or build unhealthy relationships. It is inevitable that our health may go off track at some point. Living inside the Health Matrix empowers us to identify potential risks early, take action to address them before they worsen, and get ourselves back on track across the three health dimensions. Most importantly, we are not alone on this journey, thanks to our doctors, interventionists, and health keepers.

Living Inside the Health Matrix gives us more opportunities to thrive as individuals, and it offers a better chance of living a healthier life. We don't need to depend solely on willpower when we build this matrix into our daily lives. When we know that others are there to support us in our health journey, we are more likely to build a healthy life with ease.

It is also our responsibility to build and maintain the Health Matrix together. Many of us will play the roles of each other's doctors, interventionists, and health keepers within the Health Matrix framework. It is our coordinated efforts that make complex health issues easier to tackle—and help us better recognize the unique health needs of every individual. We are all in this together.

When each of us is living as the healthiest version of ourselves, we are more likely to contribute to the world with our unique capabilities and talents. We all deserve access to the resources that will help us reach our fullest health potential. We all deserve to live in this world in our own way—and to be able to share with the world our strengths, wisdom, and kindness.

ACKNOWLEDGEMENTS

To Mingxiang Tang, for showing me the strength in standing my ground.

To Qifang Sun, for your unwavering and innate kindness.

ABOUT THE AUTHOR

TYLER YAQING TANG is the inventor of a patented preventative health delivery system that redefines how patients and health professionals work together to achieve lifelong wellbeing. As a public health innovator and research administrator, he has worked for over a decade at the intersection of health system development, patient empowerment, and equitable care design. His personal mission is to help individuals and communities thrive physically, mentally, and socially—without burning out or falling behind. Despite his pursuit of a healthier life for human beings, his three tortoises may still outlive him.

www.ingramcontent.com/pod-product-compliance
Lightning Source LLC
Chambersburg PA
CBHW032118280326
41933CB00009B/887